Model of the Etheric Physiological Structure of the Body

BAKO T.U.

GABRIELYAN S.G.

Articles collection

UDC 573.01

The collection includes the following additions articles:

Bako T.U., Gabrielyan S.G. The model of an Etherial – Physiological Structure of the Organism. Parts 1, 2. Information technologies and management. Academy of Engineering of Armenia. №№ 2-2,3, 2003. (VINITI Abstracts Journal, №4, 2005).

Bako T.U., Gabrielyan S.G. Graphical model of the system of acupuncture channels. Communications 1-5, Medical Science of Armenia. NAS RA, Vol. XLV, №№ 2,4, 2005, Vol. XLVI, №№ 1,2,3, 2006.

Bako T.U., Gabrielyan S.G. Model of Chakras System. Chakras and Acupuncture Channels. Reflexotherapy and Complementary Medicine. Science Practice Magazine, SP "Professional Association of Reflexotherapeutists", № 2(8) 2014.

Model of the Etheric Physiological Structure of the Body is presented in 2 parts:
1. A Common Theory of Oriental Medicine. An Integral Model for the System of Acupuncture Channels.

A Common Theory of Chinese, Indian and Iranian medicines is presented on the basis of a model for the system of acupuncture channels. Applying the graphic description method to the system reveals new additional functional links; in particular, 4 new extra channels and plausible master points for their activation.

2. Model of Chakras System. Chakras and Acupuncture Channels.

Model of Chakras System is related to the intercommunication between central (chakras system) and peripheral (meridians system) parts of the *thin body* (the concept of Oriental doctrine). The model describes electric processes that occur within the *thin (etheric) body* to form Sushumna and to determine the forms of spinal brain and spinal cord.

Is addressed to specialists of oriental medicine, biophysics, physicians practicing acupuncture, medical university students.

www.becomodel.com

CONTENTS

PART 1

A COMMON THEORY OF ORIENTAL MEDICINE. AN INTEGRAL MODEL FOR THE SYSTEM OF ACUPUNCTURE CHANNELS

The proposed model combines the fundamental theories of Chinese, Indian and Iranian medical traditions into an integral theoretical system.

The model graphically describes functional-energetic connections of the acupuncture meridians and predicts the presence of new additional links between them.

In this study we show that in the system of acupuncture channels there are 2 types of multifunctional groupings of the 12 classic meridians: one corresponding to 3 doshas (*pneuma, phlegm and bile*) of Indian and Tibetan medicines, and the other one corresponding to 4 primary matters (*yellow bile - safra, black bile - soda, phlegm and blood*) of Greek, Arabic and Iranian medicines.
The functional-energetic connections of the acupuncture channels are regarded as the types of integration of these 3 or 4 groupings into one energosystem. Applying this model to the system of extraordinary channels reveals 4 new extraordinary meridians and plausible master points for their activation.

The model is based on Tibetan medical science and does not contradict the theory of Chinese medicine, but supplements it by embracing the links described in other ancient medical traditions and providing, therefore, an integral concept for the energetic connections within the system.

1. THE 'MISSING' EXTRAORDINARY MERIDIANS

The suggested integral model of the meridian system stems from the Energy Circulation Cycle (Fig. 1) as it is accepted by the traditional Chinese Medicine (*Wei* level).

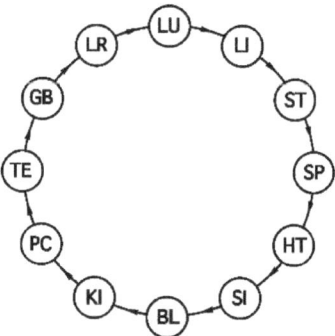

Fig.1. Energy Circulation Cycle

Several subsequent modifications of the Energy Circulation Cycle provide a graphic base for what we called Transformed Energy Circulation Cycle (TECC). To achieve that we first marked all the *yin* meridians with dark-coloured tones, and all the *yang* meridians with light-coloured tones (Fig. 2A). Then we joined the coupled meridians together (Fig. 2B) and placed them along the cycle so that all the *yang* meridians were outside, and all the *yin* meridians were inside the cycle (Fig. 2C). The resulted in transformed image of the Energy Circulation Cycle consisted of six groups of coupled meridians. It should be noted that there is no fundamental difference between TECC (Fig. 2C) and the classical way of depicting the Energy Circulation Cycle (Fig. 1).

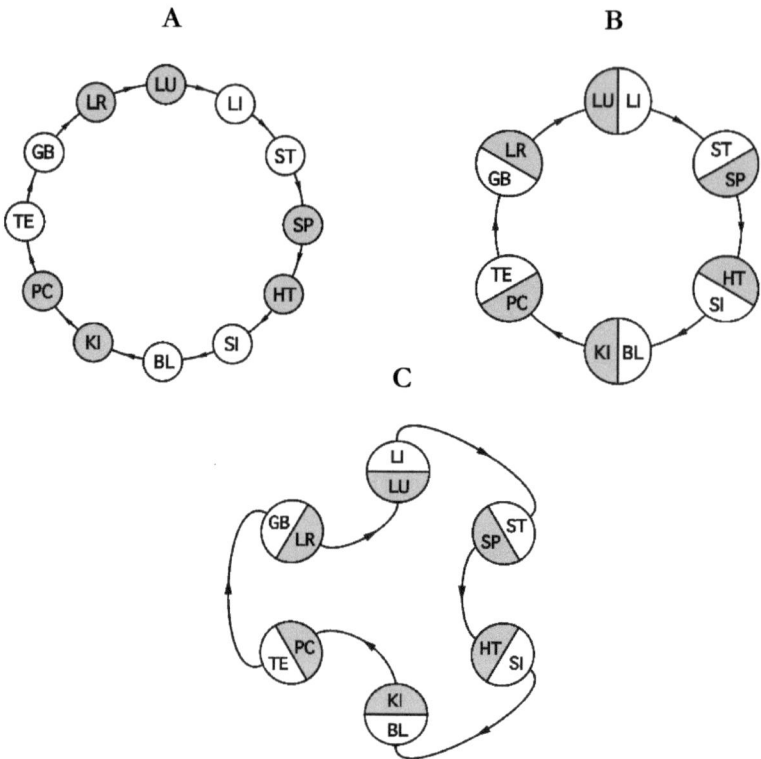

Fig. 2. Transformation of Energy Circulation Circle

We can use TECC as a platform to follow up all the known connections between the meridians. This can be done by applying one simple principle: any link between meridians is to be shown as a line, straight or curved.

For example, Fig. 3 shows three pairs of Hand-Foot *yang* meridians and three pairs of Hand-Foot *yin* meridians (Table 1) [4, 7, 10].

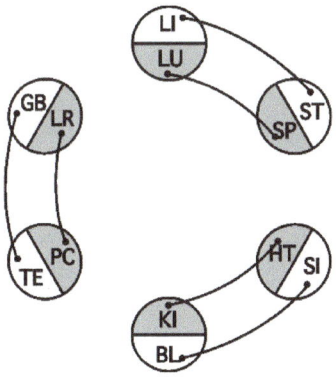

Fig. 3. 6 Big Meridians

Table 1. 6 Principal Meridians

Connection of meridians	Point of connection	Graphic designation of connection – *line*
Small intestine Bladder	BL 1	*SI – Bl*
Large intestine Stomach	ST 1	*LI – ST*
Gall bladder Three heaters	HT 21	*GB – HT*
Spleen Lungs	CV 12	*SP – LU*
Liver Pericardium	CV 18	*LR – PC*
Heart Kidney	CV 23	*HT – KI*

Similar representations can be made for other system connections. The law of midday-midnight states that in each 24-hour period each official (meridian) has a period of 2 hours when it is at its maximum energy.

Fig. 4 illustrates the meridian connections according to the law of midday-midnight (Table 2).

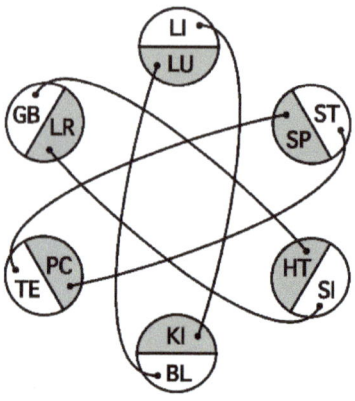

Fig. 4. Meridians Connected by 'Midday-Midnight' Law

Table 2. Meridians Connected by 'Midday-Midnight' Law

Meridians	Hrs. of max activity	Graphic designation of connection - line
Lungs Bladder	3 - 5 15 – 17	LU – BL
Large intestine Kidney	5 - 7 17 – 19	LI – KI
Stomach Pericardium	7 - 9 19 – 21	ST – PC
Spleen Three heaters	9 - 11 21 – 23	SP – HT
Heart Gall bladder	11 - 13 23 – 1	HT – GB
Small intestine Liver	13 - 15 1 – 3	SI - LR

Another example of meridian grouping is via meeting points [4, 7] connecting three upper yin meridians, three upper yang meridians, three lower yin meridians and three lower yang meridians (Fig. 5; Table 3).

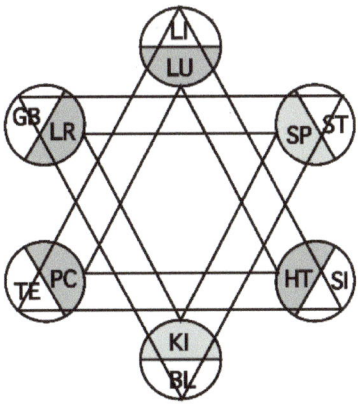

Fig. 5. Groupings of Hand and Foot (upper and lower) Meridians

Table 3. Groupings of hand and foot meridians

Meridians	Group lo-point	Graphic designation of connection - triangle
Lungs Heart Pericardium	PC 5	*LU - HT - PC*
Liver Spleen Kidney	SP 6	*LR -SP – KI*
Large intestine Small intestine Three heaters	TE 8	*LI - SI – TE*
Gall bladder Stomach Bladder	GB 39	*GB - ST – BL*

When we applied our graphic model of the meridian connections to extraordinary vessels two additional pairs of extraordinary meridians emerged from the picture. In other words, we found two 'missing' links within the system. There are 8 known extraordinary vessels [4, 6, 7, 10]. Each of these meridians has an opening point or a master point, and a coupling point which connect the extraordinary meridians into pairs (Table 4A).

Table 4A. 8 Extraordinary meridians

Group	Pair	Extraordinary meridians	Master point	Graphic designation of connection - line
I	I	Du mai Yang-chiao mai	SI 3 BL 62	*SI - BL*
	II	Yang-wei mai Dai mai	TE 5 GB 41	*TE - GB*
II	III	Ren mai Yin-chiao mai	LU 7 KI 6	*LU - KI*
	IV	Yin-wai mai Chong mai	PC 6 SP 4	*PC - SP*

If we look at all the diagrams described above (Fig. 3–5) we can see that all the links on them are symmetrical. When we transfer the known connections between the extraordinary meridians onto our graphic model (Fig. 6A) an unusual asymmetry catches the eye, and the possibility of existence of 2 more meridian pairs becomes apparent (Fig. 6B; Table 4B).

It is to be noted that the all known master points are located on the eight main meridians. A fundamental question arises: why cannot the remaining four channels carry similar key points? To find out what are the master points of the new extraordinary meridians we made the following observations:

1) all known master points are located on the 8 main meridians
2) 4 out of 8 known master points are junction points
3) the other 4 points are anatomically located between the junction points and the phalanx of toes or fingers
4) none of the known master points are source sedation points [4,7].

Taken together these observations suggest the following plausible master points for the new meridians:

on the Heart channel – HT 5 or HT 8
on the Liver channel – LR 4
on the Large Intestine channel – LI 3, LI 5 or LI 6
on the Stomach channel – ST 41 or ST 43.

A   **B**

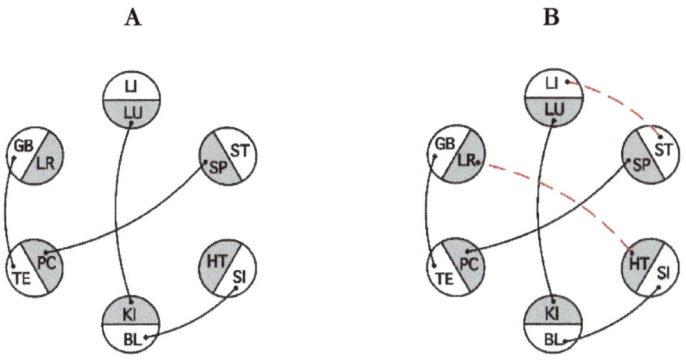

Fig. 6. 'Missing' Extraordinary Meridians

Table 4B. 12 extraordinary meridians

Group	Pair	Extraordinary meridians	Master point	Graphic designation of connection – line
I	I	Du mai Yang-chiao mai	SI 3 BL 62	*SI - BL*
	II	Yang-wei mai Dai mai	TE 5 GB 41	*TE – GB*
	V		LI 3, 5, 6 ST 41, 43	*LI – ST*
II	III	Ren mai Yin-chiao mai	LU 7 KI 6	*LU – KI*
	IV	Yin-wei mai Chong mai	PC 6 SP 4	*PC – SP*
	VI		LR 4 HT 5, 8	*LR – HT*

2. 12 MERIDIANS AND 3 DOSHAS

The theory of three vital energies or 3 *doshas (pneuma phlegm* and *bile)* constitutes the basics of Indian Ayurvedic Medicine. In Ayurveda, elements of the body are divided into 2 groups : causing disease and subjected to disease. The first group involves 7 main components of the body : <u>nutritious</u> juice – end product of food digestion, blood, muscles, fat tissues, bones, bone brain, semen and 3 products of secretion - sweat, urine, excrements. The second group involves 3 vital energies called *pneuma phlegm* and *bile.* These 2 groups of elements are mutually adjusting. If 3 vital energies are in balance, the organism is healthy. Any infraction of the balance caused by different reasons, may result in unhealthy expressions that can be seen as changes in the strength of the body (components of body) and it's debris (products of secretion) [1,3,9].

The functional activity of *pneuma* (Tibetan rlung) described as follows: "... it helps breathing and movement of seven major powers of the body, clarifying of feelings and sensations limited impact on the physical condition of the body ...". *Bile* (Tibetan mkhris) is characterized as follows: "Mkhris is located exclusively in the blood and sweat. It promotes digestion, separates nutrient juice and debris. Located in close contact with the bodily heat, gives the basis for the forces ... promotes clarity of mind and activity, and generates consciousness, intelligence, desire ... makes it possible to see the images of objects, produces a distinct clarity in the color of the skin. " Functions of *phlegm* (Tibetan Bad-kan) relate to the regulation of body water, all the diseases that occur on a background of obesity and joint damage [3]. The following quotation from "Chzhud-shek" Wind and Mucus match *pneuma*, and *phlegm*. "The Wind shall breathe in and out, gives the force that causes the body in motion, direct the movement of physical forces within the body, makes clear the senses and leads the body. Bile depends on the feeling of hunger and thirst, feeding, digestion, bodily warmth, color, courage and intelligence, Mucus enhances the body and mind, gives a dream. It is responsible for joints, soft and oily body" [9]. Each of the three physiological energies exist as five currents that perform specific functions.

What are the three doshas? Their characteristics cited in ancient medical treatises give rise to different interpretations. Authors of scientific project, devoted to Tibetan medicine based on relevance of Tibetan and modern information on ways of organism regulation came to the following conclusion : ".. the key moment to determine the system of regulation in Tibetan medicine is the way of regulatory signal transfer ". There are 3 systems of regulations to be considered based on this criteria – wind, bile and mucus, that we identify as neural, humoral and local tissue ways of regulation respectively [8]. Local tissue or diffuse neuro-endocrine system, the latter being peptide-secreting cells diffusively scattered in the viscera and in brain tissues and producing the regulatory peptides [5].

Our clue to this problem is the following quotation from the Medieval Tibetan treatise "The Blue Beryl" (Atlas of Tibetan Medicine.)

According to *Blue Beryl*: "These vessels consist of Four vessels of *pneuma* connecting Heart and Small intestine, four vessels of *bile* connecting Lungs, Large Intestine, Liver and Gall Bladder, four vessels of *phlegm* connecting Stomach, Spleen, Kidneys and Bladder' [2].

Note that in Oriental sources "vessel" term means not only blood vessels and nerve plexus, but also different invisible energy currents-channels of the *thin body* that maintain life and organism development in general. *

---

* Oriental philosophy medical teachings present the human body as a combination of 3 bodies : root body, thin body and dense or rough body. The root body or the body of semen – is bodiless Spirit that enters the womb at the moment of conceiving and starts embryo development. It will generate thin and rough bodies later on.

As known, Tibetan medicine was formed approximately in VII century by acknowledgement of ancient experience and knowledge of traditions of India, China and Iran, that have been combined into one system. The process of thousand years of development of Tibetan medicine also assumed the fusion of different theory concepts. Having discovered the functional links of vital origins of *pneuma, bile* and *phlegm* with hollow and dense organs (as cited), Tibetan medics could establish the relevance between fundamental concepts of Indian and Chinese schools. This became a foundation for integrated theory of oriental medicine that has not been developed further. By using experiences of Tibetan medical scientists that would see vital energies are groupings of *organs*, we suggest to develop this theory by considering 3 vital origins as functional groupings of 12 main meridians. There are 3 possible variants of grouping with 3 axes of symmetry, positioned in relation to each other under 120° angle:

1.   LI-LU-BL-KI,   SI-HT-GB-LR,   TE-PC-ST-SP
2.   LI-LU-ST-SP,   SI-HT-BL-KI,   TE-PC-GB-LR
3.   LI-LU-GB-LR,   SI-HT-ST-SP,   TE-PC-BL-K.

Our model suggests that only the third combination (Fig. 7) proves to be functional.

Table 5

	Bile	**Phlegm**	**Pneuma**
Tratise *Blue Beryl*	LI - LU - GB – LR	BL - KI - ST - SP	SI – HT
Suggested model	LI - LU - GB – LR	BL - KI - TE - PC	SI - HT - ST - SP

Thin body that appears within 2 months of embryo development consists of numeral invisible vessels (channels) with circulating life energy. There are 3 vessels called forming that appear the first in the developing embryo. The main vessel- flow goes from head to sexual organs. The other 2 forming vessels go close to the right and left sides of the central vessel. The 3 forming vessels cross each other and make branches to create chakras. As a result a net of smaller vessels (managing vessels) appears around chakras , that are responsible for functionality of sense organs, "generating 6 kinds of sensual comprehension", responsible for regeneration etc. [1].

Note that *bile* in our model is identical to the variant of Tibetan medics. As cited, the Chinese theory speaks only about 10 main *organs*, and 2 others, Three heaters and Pericardium – had not yet been added , although they have been discovered later. Much probably it is for this reason that the other two groups are not absolutely identical to *phlegm* and *pneuma*.

3 groups, corresponding to physiological principles, are formed in the further transformation of the Energy Circulation Cycle (Fig. 7 A,B,C). Let's illustrate the above presented functional links (Fig. 3 - 6) onto new graphic basis (Fig. 7C).

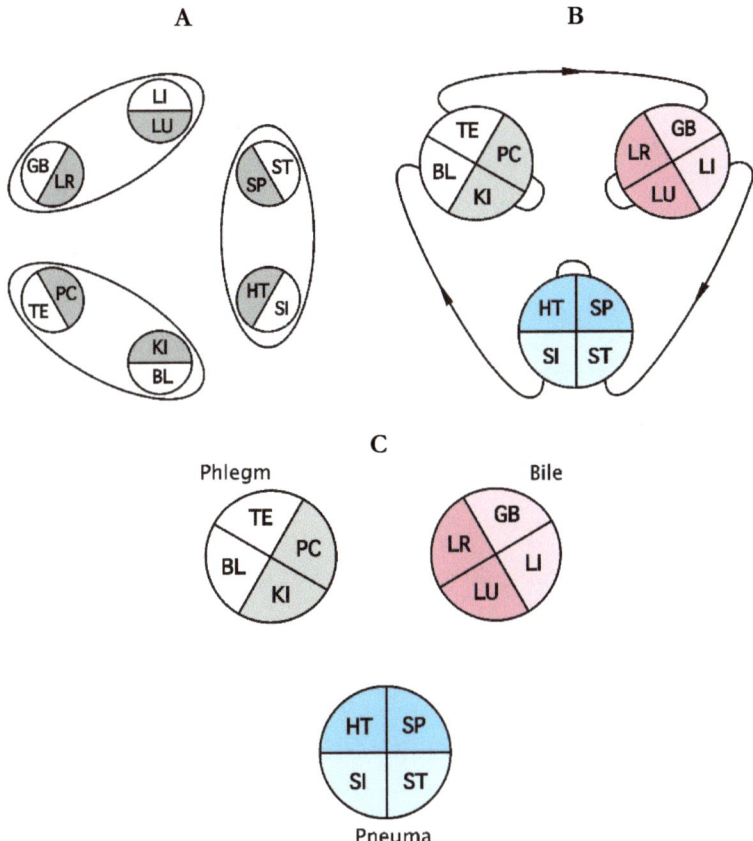

Fig. 7. 3 groupings of 12 meridians

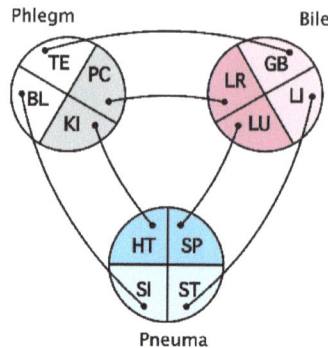

Fig. 8. 6 Big Meridians

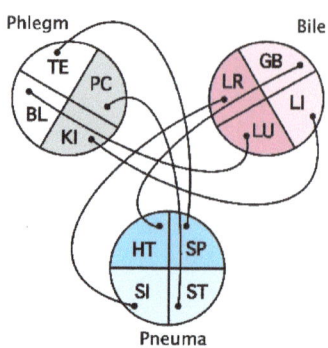

Fig. 9. Meridians Connected by
'Midday- Midnight' Law

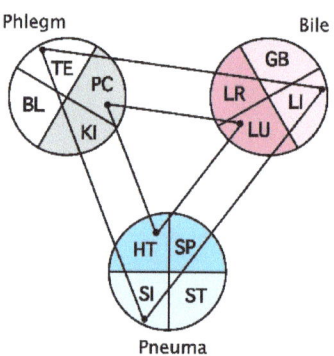

Fig. 10. Groupings of Hand and Foot (upper and lower) Meridians

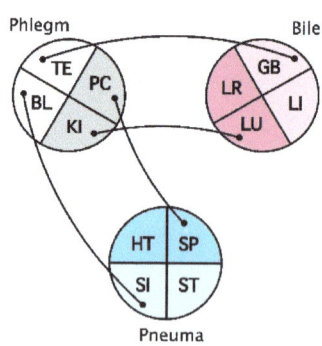

Fig. 11. 4 pairs of
Extraordinary Meridians

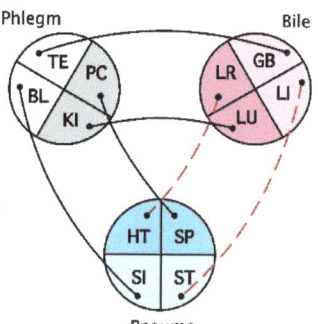

Fig. 12. 6 pairs of
Extraordinary Meridians

Obviously, the 6 Big meridians, meridians connected by 'Midday - Midnight' law and groups of hand and foot meridians, form a closed system, connecting with each other *phlegm*, *bile* and *pneuma* (Fig.8-10), and in case of extraordinary meridians there are missing links between *bile* and *pneuma* (Fig. 11). This way, another 2 new pairs of extraordinary meridians have been discovered (Fig. 12, Table 4B).

3. CONNECTIONS BY ANALOGY

When we transfer all the types of meridian connections considered above on one graphic base which shows the links between three doshas we can see that *phlegm*, *bile* and *pneuma* connect to each other in 3 different ways:

  a) via yin meridians (Fig. 13, Fig. 14 A,B),
  b) via yang meridians (Fig. 13, Fig. 14 A,B),
  c) via yin-yang meridians (Fig. 14C).

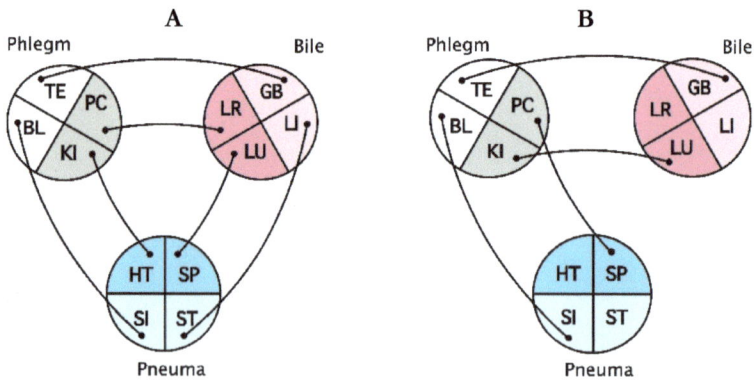

Fig.13. Connections between 3 Doshas via 6 Big (A) and Extraordinary Meridians (B)

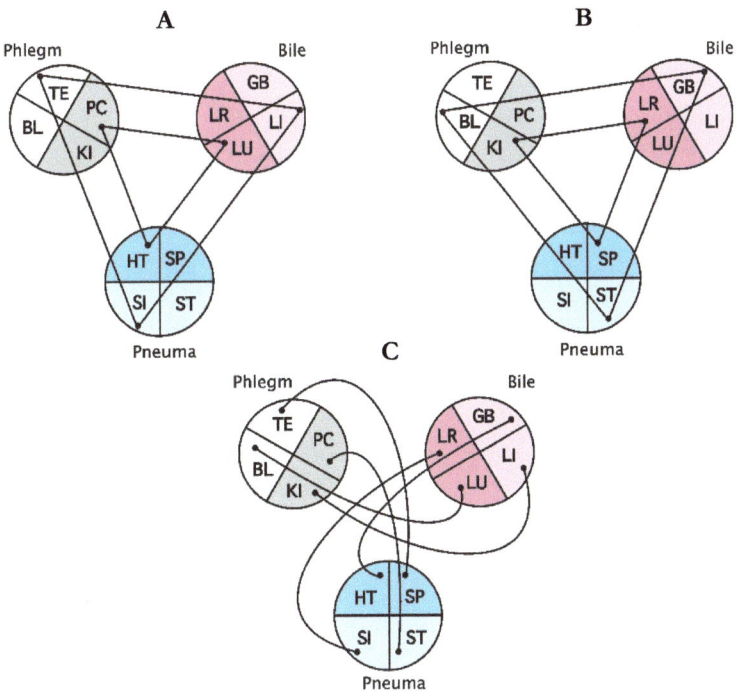

Fig. 14. Connections between 3 Doshas via Hand (A) and Foot (B) Groupings, and According to the Law of ' Midday-Midnight' (C)

Let's analyse these connections using as examples PC and TE meridians.

a) Connections via yin meridians (Fig. 15A).

The line PC–LR is Jueyin meridian (Fig. 13A), the line PC–SP is pair IV of Extraordinary meridians Yin Wei Mai and Chong Mai (Fig. 13B) and the two lines PC–HT and PC–LU are part of the functional grouping of hand yin meridians (Fig. 14A,B). In this example *phlegm* is communicating with *bile* and *pneuma* in 4 different ways.

b) Connections via yang meridians (Fig. 15B).

The line TE–GB represents both Shaoyang meridian (Fig. 13A), and pair II of Extraordinary meridians Yang Wei Mai and Dai Mai (Fig. 13B). The two lines TE–LI and TE–SI are part of the functional grouping of hand yang meridians (Fig. 14A,B).

Therefore, *phlegm* is communicating with *bile* and *pneuma* here in 3 different ways.

c)   Connections via yin-yang meridians (Fig. 15C).

There is only one way of connecting doshas via yin-yang meridians – according to the law of midday-midnight, in this example PC–ST (Fig. 14C).

This analysis reveals 'the missing links'. In the first example (Fig. 15A), two lines PC–HT and PC–LU represent connections between hand meridians, and the other two lines PC–LR and PC–SP represent connections between hand and foot meridians. In the second example (Fig. 15B), two connections are between hand meridians (TE–LI and TE–SI) and only one connection is between hand and foot meridians (TE–GB). Apparently, one connection TE–ST between hand and foot meridians is missing. In the third example (Fig. 15C), there is only one link between hand and foot meridians (line PC-ST). Since, we have not found in literature any

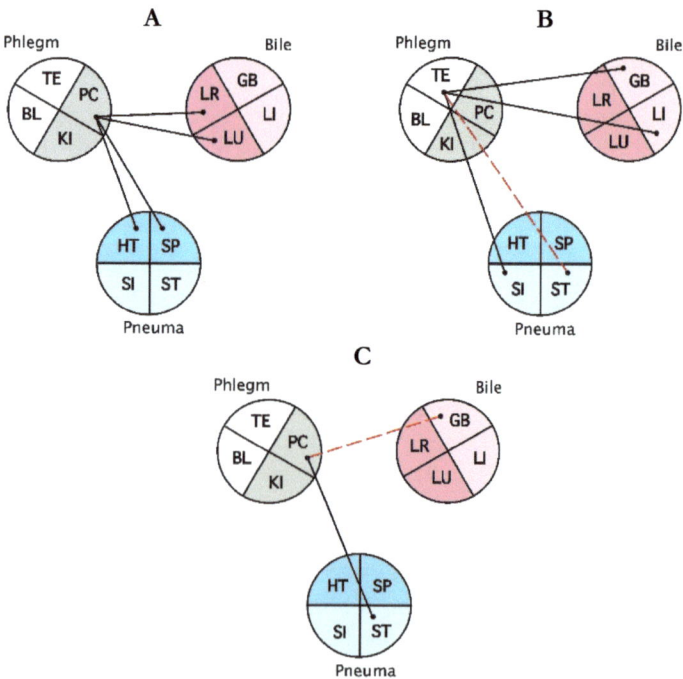

Fig. 15. Connections between 3 Doshas via yin (A), yang (B) and yin-yang (C) Meridians

description of theoretically possible connections between hand meridians PC–SI and PC–LI, we would refrain from including them in the list of suggested connections and would confine to PC–GB type connections between foot and hand meridians by analogy with PC–ST. Suggested new TE–ST and PC–GB connections are shown in Fig. 18A, B and Fig. 18C, respectively.

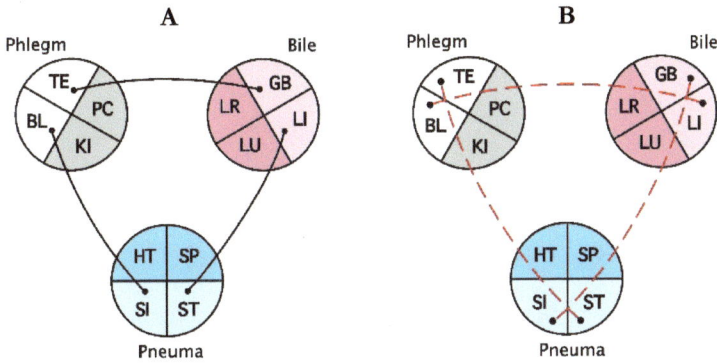

Fig. 16. Connections between 3 Doshas via yang Meridians

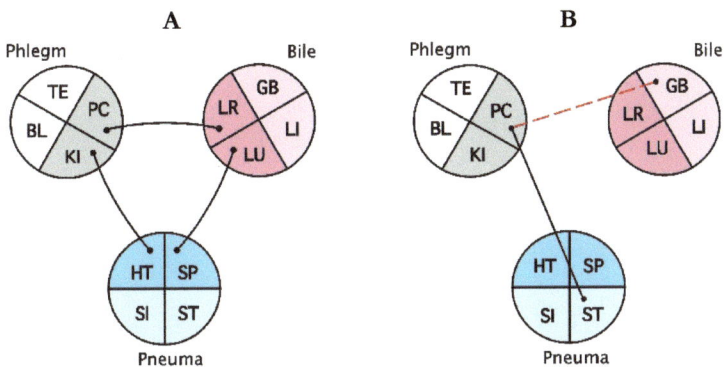

Fig. 17. Connections between 3 Doshas via yin Meridians

If we now look at all possibilities of integrating 3 doshas via hand and foot meridians, we discover 3 fundamentally different functional-energetic types of connections (Fig. 18A,B,C). Yang and yin variations are shown separately in Fig. 16 and Fig. 17.

Combining the variation shown in Fig. 16A with the ones shown in Fig. 17A and Fig. 17B results in the Big meridians (Fig. 13A), and the Extraordinary meridians (Fig. 13C), respectively. Two other combinations, Fig. 16B with Fig. 17A and Fig. 16B with Fig. 17B, reveal two fundamentally different types of interactions, which we called connections by analogy with 6 Big meridians (Fig. 17A) and connections by analogy with extraordinary meridians (Fig. 18B). Fig.18C illustrates the connections by analogy with 'midday-midnight' law.

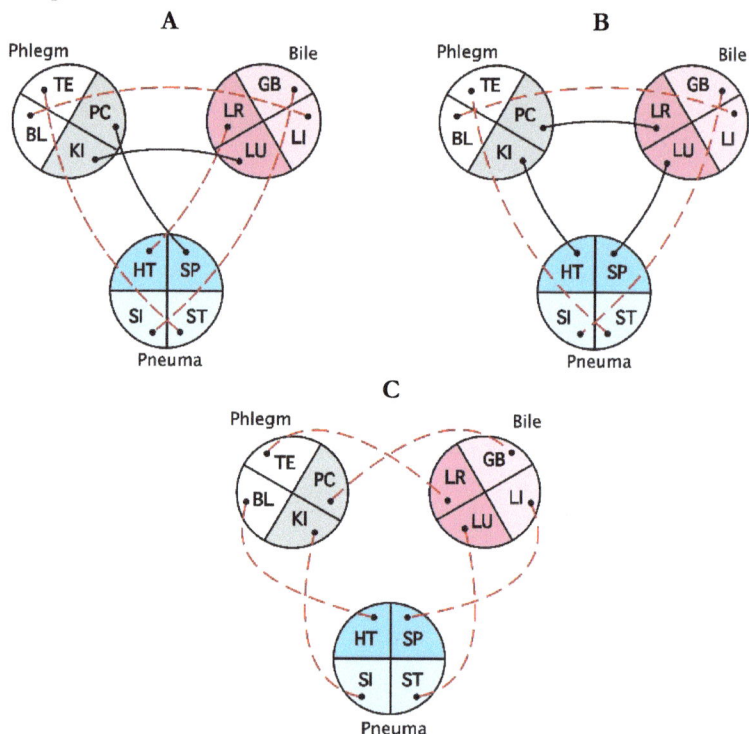

Fig. 18. Connections between 3 Doshas by Analogy with 6 Big (A) and Extraordinary Meridians (B) and the 'Midday-Midnight' Law (C)

All the connections described above are summarized in Table 6.

Table 6. Types of Connections between the Three Doshas

Types of Connections		Graphic Images of Connections between		
		Phlegm and Pneuma	Phlegm and Bile	Bile and Pneuma
		Lines		
I	6 Big Principal Meridians	BL -SI KI - HT	TE – GB PC – LR	LI – ST LU - SP
	Connections by Analogy with the 6 Big Principal Meridians	TE - ST PC - SP	BL – LI KI – LU	GB – ST LR - HT
II	Extraordinary Meridians	BL - SI PC - SP	TE – GB KI – LU	LI - ST LR - HT
	Connections by Analogy with Extraordinary Meridians	TE – ST KI – HT	BL - LI PC – LR	GB - SI LU – SP
III	"Midday – Midnight" Law	TE - SP PC - ST	BL – LU KI – LI	GB – HT LR - SI
	Connections by Analogy with "Midday – Midnight" Law	BL - HT KI - SI	TE – LR PC – GB	LI – SP LU - ST
IV	Groupings of Hand Meridians	BL - ST KI - SP	BL – GB KI – LR	GB – ST LR - SP
	Groupings of Foot Meridians	TE - SI PC - HT	TE – LI PC – LU	LI – SI LU - HT

19

4. 12 MERIDIANS AND 4 MATTERS OF THE BODY

The fundamental idea of ancient natural philosophy about proto-substances or basic elements of nature – Air, Fire, Water and Earth – constitutes the core of the Greek, Arabic and Iranian medical systems. Each of these 4 elements is described as having certain qualities: Air is hot and damp, Fire is hot and dry, Water is cold and damp, and Earth is cold and dry. According to the Greek-Iranian-Arabic medical school, the human body also contains 4 different matters matching the 4 elements: *blood* is by nature similar to Air (hot and damp), *safra (yellow bile)* is similar to Fire, *phlegm* is similar to Water, and *soda (black bile)* – is similar to Earth. Those matters are produced during the assimilation or conversion of food. The first stage of assimilation starts while chewing the food in the mouth, where from it goes as mushy substance into the stomach, whereas the more consistent part of that mush (excretions) goes to the intestine. Stage 2 is occurring in the liver receiving the liquid of the mush via the vessels allegedly linking stomach with liver. The products of this assimilation stage are basic liquid substances: *blood, safra, soda and phlegm* which further proceed to the intestine, while the waste (urine) is removed through kidneys and the urinary bladder. Stage 3 of the conversion is occurring in the vessels. At this stage the 4 basic liquid substances are converted into components of tissues and organs. Conversion of food is completed within organs and tissues (stage 4) by production of substances similar to the substances of the organs. The waste from this stage, which is sweat and fat, is removed through skin cover.

In pursuance to this medical tradition, the human nature (*mizoj*– merge) is determined by mixing the liquid substances occurring at stage 3 of food conversion, their ratios being determinant of the type of temper. There are 9 types of living creatures and organisms: 4 simple natures with the prevalence of heat, cold, dryness, moisture; 4 compound natures with the prevalence of heat and moisture, heat and dryness, cold and moisture, cold and dryness and 1 rarely occurring type of the *truly balanced nature.*

This principle adopted by the European medicine persisted throughout the Middle Age and into the Renaissance. According to it, sanguines (Sanguis – *blood*) are personalities with dominating *blood* qualities (heat and dampness), cholerics (Kholê – *bilè*) are personalities with dominating *safra*, phlegmatics (*phlegm*) are the ones with dominating *phlegm*, and melancholics (Melancholia – *black bilè*) are the ones with dominating *soda* [5]. The differences in personalities are taken into account in the treatment of patients.

In the East, astrology was an accepted scientific discipline from the ancient times, the concept of proto substances (elements) being a part of it. In the zodiac circle each of the four elements is presented as a triangle (trigon) (Fig. 19), which includes 3 zodiac signs. It determines the character of a person born under particular zodiac sign, as well as the possible pathologies in their body, and imbalances in their energy channels.

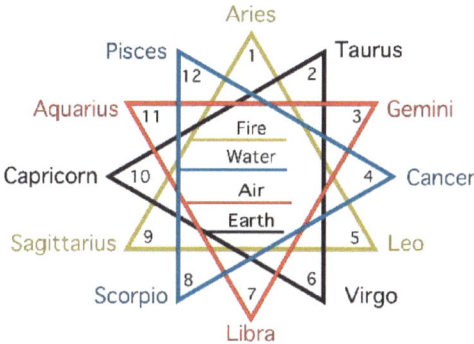

Fig. 19. The Band of Zodiak

The Table 7 shows zodiac signs correspondences to the basic meridians.

Table 7. Relevance of Zodiac signs to 12 meridians

Zodiac sign		Variations											
		1	2	3	4	5	6	7	8	9	10	11	12
1	Aries	LU	LI	ST	SP	HT	SI	BL	KI	PC	TE	GB	LR
2	Taurus	LI	ST	SP	HT	SI	BL	KI	PC	TE	GB	LR	LU
3	Gemini	ST	SP	HT	SI	BL	KI	PC	TE	GB	LR	LU	LI
4	Cancer	SP	HT	SI	BL	KI	PC	TE	GB	LR	LU	LI	ST
5	Leo	HT	SI	BL	KI	PC	TE	GB	LR	LU	LI	ST	SP
6	Virgo	SI	BL	KI	PC	TE	GB	LR	LU	LI	ST	SP	HT
7	Libra	BL	KI	PC	TE	GB	LR	LU	LI	ST	SP	HT	SI
8	Scorpio	KI	PC	TE	GB	LR	LU	LI	ST	SP	HT	SI	BL
9	Sagittarius	PC	TE	GB	LR	LU	LI	ST	SP	HT	SI	BL	KI
10	Capricorn	TE	GB	LR	LU	LI	ST	SP	HT	SI	BL	KI	PC
11	Aquarius	GB	LR	LU	LI	ST	SP	HT	SI	BL	KI	PC	TE
12	Pisces	LR	LU	LI	ST	SP	HT	SI	BL	KI	PC	TE	GB

Trigon of Fire consists of Aries, Leo and Sagittarius, that is 1, 5 and 9 signs of Zodiac (Fig.19). Let's investigate the relevance of Fire to 12 main meridians (Table 8).

Table 8. Relevance Variations of Fire and 12 meridians

FIRE	Variations											
	1	2	3	4	5	6	7	8	9	10	11	12
Aries	LU	LI	ST	SP	HT	SI	BL	KI	PC	TE	GB	LR
Leo	HT	SI	BL	KI	PC	TE	GB	LR	LU	LI	ST	SP
Sagittarius	PC	TE	GB	LR	LU	LI	ST	SP	HT	SI	BL	KI

Let's pay our attention to the fact that 1, 5, and 9 variations are identical, they consists of the same meridians (lungs, heart, pericardium), that have different combinations in each variation. There are also other variations that are identical as 2, 6, 10 (LI–SI–TE); 3, 7, 11 (ST-BL–GB) и 4, 8, 12 (SP-KI–LR). We can see that these combinations are relevant to functional groupings of hand and foot meridians. (Fig. 5) (Table 3).

Table 9. Astrological and biological aspects of the four proto substances

Element	Matter of the body	Grouping of meridians			
		Variations			
		1	2	3	4
FIRE	Yellow Bile	Large intestine Small intestine Three heaters SI - LI - TE	Liver Spleen Kidney LR - SP - KI	Lungs Heart Pericardium LU - HT- PC	Gall bladder Stomach Bladder GB- ST - BL
WATER	Phlegm	Gall bladder Stomach Bladder GB - ST - BL	Lungs Heart Pericardium LU - HT- PC	Large intestine Small intestine Three heaters SI - LI - TE	Liver Spleen Kidney LR - SP - KI
EARTH	**Black Bile**	Liver Spleen Kidney LR - SP - KI	Large intestine Small intestine Three heaters SI - LI - TE	Gall bladder Stomach Bladder GB - ST - BL	Lungs Heart Pericardium LU - HT- PC
AIR	Blood	Lungs Heart Pericardium LU - HT- PC	Gall bladder Stomach Bladder GB - ST- BL	Liver Spleen Kidney LR - SP - KI	Large intestine Small intestine Three heaters SI - LI - TE

A biological analog of Fire is *yellow bile* (*safra*) [5]. Therefore, *yellow bile* is relevant to one of these 4 groups : 3 hand yin (LU - HT - PC), 3 hand yang (LI - SI - TE), 3 foot yin (LR -SP - KI) or 3 foot yang (GB - ST - BL) meridians. We same picture can be seen for trigons of Water, Earth and Air (Table 9). Therefore, '4 matters of the body' represent the links between hand and foot meridians.

REFERENCES

1. Atlas of Tibetan Medicine. Collection of illustrations to the medical treatise of 17 century. 1998 (in Russian).
2. Atlas of Tibetan Medicine. Collection of illustrations to the medical treatise of 17 century. p. 120, 1998 (in Russian).
3. Bazaron EG, Aseeva TA,"Vaidurya-onbo" - a treatise of the Indo-Tibetan Medicine. 1984 (in Russian).
4. G.Luvsan. Traditional and Modern Aspects of Oriental Reflex therapy. 1986 (in Russian).
5. The wisdom of centuries. Ancient medicine about health reservation. 1991 (in Russian).
6. Nguen Van Hghi .Traditional Chinese medicine. Pathogenesis of diseases. Diagnostics. Therapy. 2000 (in Russian).
7. Tabeeva D.M Guide on reflex-therapy. 1980 (in Russian).
8. Hundanov LL, Batomunkueva TV, Hundanova LL. Tibetan Medicine. 1993 (in Russian).
9. "Chzhud-shek" - a monument of medieval Tibetan culture. 1988 (in Russian).
10. Shnorrenberger C. Textbook of Chinese medicine to Western physicians. 1996 (in Russian).

PART 2

MODEL OF CHAKRAS SYSTEM.
CHAKRAS AND ACUPUNCTURE CHANNELS

The second part of a *Model of the Etheric Physiological Structure of the body* is related to the intercommunication between central and peripheral parts of the *thin body* (the concept of Oriental doctrine) that is between chakras and meridians thanks to discovery of 3 yin and 3 yang chakras.

The proposed model describes electric processes that occur within the *thin (etheric) body* to form Sushumna (chakras, Chitrini and Vajra nadis) and to determine the forms of spinal brain and spinal cord.

It is assumed that recognizing the regularities of energy distribution in the chakras and determination of those systems functional interdependencies can become a fundamental principle for deploying new methods of healing upon the individual frequency characteristics of the organism.

INTRODUCTION

According to philosophy of yoga man is a microcosm that fully reflects the life of macrocosm and by knowing oneself one is able to recognize the true reality of Universe. In theology this reality is determined as Spirit (Pure Consciousness) from which through its force (Shakti) or dynamic aspect of Spirit all the creative expressions of Universe have been originated.

According to this teaching, it is possible to achieve the highest existence by connecting or merging human personality with Universe Consciousness.

The process of yoga assumes the expansion of level of Consciousness that leads to opening of inner substance of man which is Pure Consciousness ; and all the forms of yoga (hatha yoga, radja yoga, jnana yoga etc) – are different methods of spiritual practice leading to this cherished target.

Kundalini- yoga is a special form of tantric yoga where yoga is being exposed by penetrating into 6 centers of body (lotos or chakras (circle or ring - sancsript)) of cosmic force of Kundalini (curved into ring - sanscripts). This force is described as Pure Consciousness, the primary Nature (Prakriti), "Spritual force " etc. This very force "maintains all beings of the world by means of inspiration and expiration".

Creative force of Kundalini-Shakti in the human body is symbolically pictured as a snake that is napping in the lower center of Muladhara chakra. After wakening she goes up to connect with

Shiva (static aspect of Universe Consciousness), which is being exposed in the highest brain center of Sahasrara lotus. Upon this rise Kundalini activates chakras that are located along the spinal cord. The most detailed teaching of charkras is represented in *Sat-Chakra-Nirupana* written in XVI century by Purananda Swami. According to this source, there are 6 main chakras:

> Muladhara (mula – root, dhara – base);
> Svadhisthana (sweetness, one's own dwelling place);
> Manipura ("resplendent gem ", city of gemstones);
> Anahata ("unstruck" or "unhurt");
> Vishuddha (pure, clean);
> Ajna (to know, to recognize, to command) and
> brain center Sahasrara (thousand petaled).

Traditionally chakras are related to nerve plexus and endocrine glands. However, despite an amazing correspondence of formal description of the given system with anatomic location of nerve plexus, and also correspondence of their mental characteristics with psychic functions and processes – it is impossible to categorize chakras in only one science discipline (physiology, psychology, philosophy etc). "To do it this way, means not only to spoil the thing, but destroy it because physiology doesn't recognize chakras, because they exist separately as the centers of Consciousness and activity of sukshma-prana-vayu or thin vital force, although they deal with rough body that is referred to them " (sir J.G.Woodroffe).

In Buddha tantras they mention 4 chakras: navel, heart, throat and brain (there are different opinions yet about the number and location of these chakras). The first 3 chakras are the locations of 3 Buddha bodies : *root , thin and dense (rough) ones*. The *root body* or the body of semen – is bodiless Spirit that enters the womb at the moment of conceiving and starts embryo development. It will generate thin and rough bodies later on. *Thin body* that appears within 2 months of embryo development consists of numeral invisible vessels (channels) with circulating life energy. There are 3 vessels called forming that appear the first in the developing embryo. The main vessel- flow goes from head to sexual organs. The other 2 forming vessels go close to the right and left sides of the central vessel. The 3 forming vessels cross each other and make branches to create chakras. As a result a net of smaller vessels (managing vessels) appears around chakras , that are responsible for functionality of sense organs, "generating 6 kinds of sensual comprehension", responsible for regeneration etc. [1]. Formation of *dense* or *rough body* is stimulated and supported by life energy of *thin body*.

From numerous vessels of *thin body* there are 3 forming vessels called Ida, Pingala and Sushumna to be the most important according to Indian tradition. Sushumna originates from the base of spine and rises up through spinal cord. In the area of middle brain (Ajna-chakra) it divides into branches that come to Brahma-randhra by different ways (this spot is associated with the top of the head and considered to be 10th gateways of the body). There are 3 nadi channels passing through Sushumna – Vajra nadi, Chitrini nadi (or Citrini nadi) and Brahma nadi. *"In varse 2 (*Sat-Chakra-Nirupana*) says that inside Vajra which itself is located inside Sushumna, there is Chitrini which is subtle as a spider's thread, and pierces all the Lotuses which are placed within the backbone. The other statement in varse 51 is a bit confusing saying that lotuses are located in/ on Brahma nadi. Vishvanandha commented this by citing Maya-Tantra and saying that all 6 lotoses are connected to Chitrini nadi. From all this it becomes apparent that lotuses are located in the spinal cord, in Sushumna, but not in surrounding nerve plexus* [2]. Sushumna is also called Brahma nadi, mahapatha (great way), shmashana (cemetery), shambhavi (one of the names of Durga), madhyaramarga (middle way). In this article we 'll use terms Brahma nadi for central channel and Sushumna for multi-layer structure.

The 2 other vessels Pingala and Ida also begin from base of spine, reaching Ajna chakra and going through nose channel ending in the left and right nostrils accordingly. There are different versions regarding their real location; some researchers state that these channels are out of Meruanda (spinal channel), the other one gives a reference to *Nigama tattva Saru* stating Ida and Pingala are inside Meru [2]. If taking into account that chakras are being created in the juncture points of 3 forming vessels and beaded on Chitrini nadi, then we should accept the logics of the second statement, that Ida and Pingala are inside the spinal cord.

Unfortunately, there is no accurate answer to the question : which origin these channels are related to, feminine or masculine one? The following citate of Arthur Avalon (Sir John Woodroffe), the translator, indicates the contradiction and undefined situation.

In the space out of Meru (spine) on the left and right there are 2 shira (nadis): Shasi (moon, t.e feminine origin or Shakti-rupa nadi ida, on the left) and Mihira (sun or masculine origin, pingala, on the right) (Satcakranirupana, 1-3; tr. Arthur Avalon, the Serpent Power. Madras, 1924, p.4 — 12.)
…According to Sammohana –tantra (citing « Shatchakranirupana »), ida is Shakti, and pingala is Purusha. In other sources they say that lalana (ida) and rasana (pingala) pass semen and egg respectively. («Sadhanamala», «Khevajra-tantra » and «Kherukta-tantra» are cited by Dasgupta, Introduction to Tantric Buddhism, p. 119.) And semen is the substance of Shiva and Moon, and menstrual blood (associated with « rajas » of women) is the substance of Shakti and sun. («Gorakshsidhantasangraha », cited by Dasgupta,p. 172). In the comments on « «Dohakosha » of Kanhupada it is said that moon was born from masculine semen, and the sun was born from egg' [3].

FORMATION OF SUSHUMNA

Chakras are symbolically described via sound vibrations (mantras), geometric figures (yantras), god, sense organs , organs of actions etc, and also through primary elements or tattvas. Each tattva has definite number of rays; from 6 chakras we have 3 groups – Fire, Sun and Moon (Table 1). In Taitirja-aranjak they say:

Devi- the cause of creation, protection and destroyment of Universe is here (Sahasrare), always connected with Sadashiva, which is the highest of all tattvas , eternally shining. Rays coming out of her body are uncountable …360 of these rays illuminate the world in the form of Fire, Sun and Moon. These 360 rays are formed as follows : Agni (Fire) 118, Sun 106, Moon 136» [2].

Table 1. Correspondence of chakras, tattvas and gunas

Chakra		Element (tattva)	Number of tattva rays	Number of group rays	Group	Guna
1	Muladhara	Earth	56	118	Fire	Tamas
2	Svadhisthana	Water	62			
3	Manipura	Fire	52	106	Sun	Radjas
4	Anahata	Air	54			
5	Visuddha	Ether	72	136	Moon	Sattva
6	Ajna	Maha-tattva	64			

Moon, Sun and Fire symbolize 3 fundamental qualities of world creation (3 gunas – sattva, radjas, tamas) [2], biological analogs of which are 3 doshas of Indian Ayurveda medicine kapha (phlegm or mucus), pitta (bile) and vayu (pneuma or wind).

Correspondence of chakras and doshas can be defined by their location, given in Tibetan treatise Chjud-shek (Table 2).

"Phlegm is standing on brain, located at the top,
bile is standing on diaphragm, located in the middle,
wind is standing on lumbus, located at the bottom" [4].

Table 2 . Correspondence of chakras and 3 doshas

	Chakra	Chakra Location	Dosha	Location of Doshas
1	Muladhara	Base of the spine	Pneuma	*wind is standing on lumbus, located at the bottom*
2	Svadhisthana	Between pubic bone and navel		
3	Manipura	Navel area	Bile	*bile is standing on diaphragm, located in the middle*
4	Anahata	Heart area		
5	Visuddha	Throat	Phlegm	*phlegma is standing on brain, located at the top*
6	Ajna	Glabella		

According to *Common theory of Oriental medicine* 3 doshas are functional groups for 12 classic meridians (Fig. 1, Table 3) [5]. Each dosha is related to 4 meridians and 2 chakras (Tables 2,3). Therefore, 1 chakra is connected with 2 acupuncture channels (meridians). In this regard there are several ways of connections available; in order to make the grounded choice let's go back to tattvas (Table 1).

Table 3. 3 doshas and 12 acupuncture channels

Dosha	Grouping of acupuncture channels
Pneuma	Small intestine, Heart, stomach, Spleen SI - HT - ST – SP
Bile	Gall bladder , Liver, Large intestine, Lungs GB - LR - LI – LU
Phlegm	Ur. Bladder , Kidney, 3 heaters, Pericardium BL -KI - TE – PC

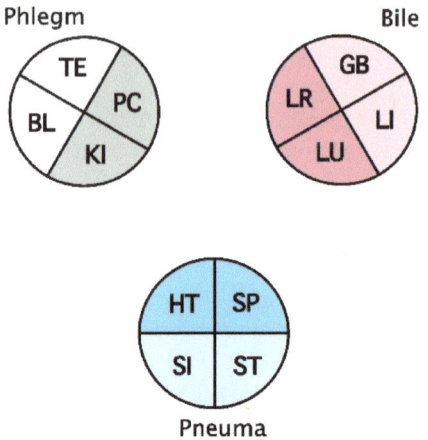

Fig. 1. 3 groups of 12 meridians

We can see that the total sum of tattva rays for 1,3, 5 chakras is equal to the sum of tattva 2,4, 6 chakras : 56+52+72 = 62+54+64 = 180. This way these 2 groups (2, 4, 6 and 1, 3, 5) with equal potential of (180), being a part of the integrity (180+180=360) are missing the sign of opposite to be considered as the concept of yin /yang. This sign is revealed further, in result of which we can represent the connection between chakras and meridians (Table 4).

According to tantras, Kundalini Shakti rises along Brahma nadi; the flow in the central channel of Sushumna is pointing up. There are 2 flows that are passing via Ida and Pingala – fresh, wet, moon flow (white), spreading the system by nectar and hot, dry, sun flow (red), which dries out all the system, moistured by nectar, that is 2 polar flows: prana and apana, one is down-top , the other is top-down. Directions of flows in 3 main vessels are the sign of electromagnet interactions between them. The graphic example is shown on Fig. 2. The core magnet NS is firmly fixed; a flexible metal pipe KA is hanged near it. Upon current passing through it the conductor is positioning at 90 angle towards magnet: the strip embraces the magnet by spirals [6]. It is not difficult to imagine that by changing the direction of the current, the strip will embrace the magnet in opposite direction as well. In this sample the vertical lines of magnet field along the NS axes are similar to Brahma nadi, and spiral conductor is similar to Ida and Pingala depending on direction of the current going through it.

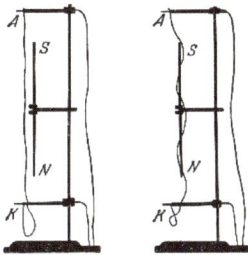

Fig. 2. Electromagnetic interaction of core magnet and conductor with current

Vectors of magnetic field tension of upward and downward currents are pointing up (Fig. 3). These currents may correspond to both Ida and Pingala. Therefore, there are 2 possible variants of the model:

1. the current of Ida is pointed down, and Pingala's – up (Fig. 3A);
2. the current of Ida is pointed up, and Pingala's - down (Fig. 3B).

In the first case the right half of the body will match Moon (Ida), and left half – Sun (Pingala). In the second case vice versa.

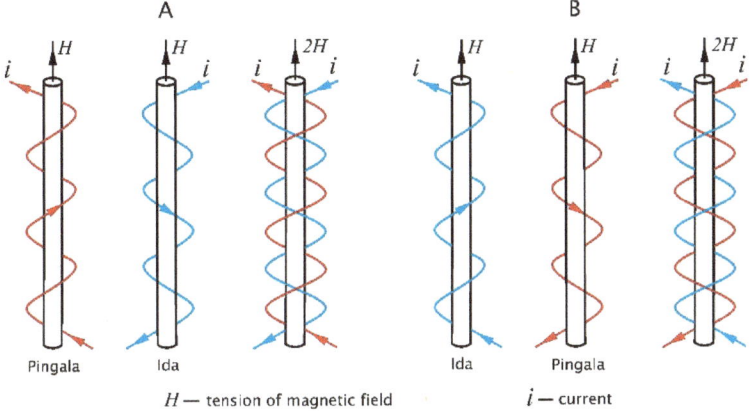

Fig. 3. Vectors of magnetic field tension of upward and downward currents

The first variant of model (considered in this article) assumes that Ida symbolizes the masculine origin, and Pingala – the feminine one. And the variant 2 – vice versa. In any case the end result as a connection of meridians and chakras is the same not depending on variations.

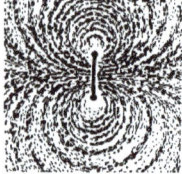

Fig. 4. Force lines of magnetic field of circuit conductor with current

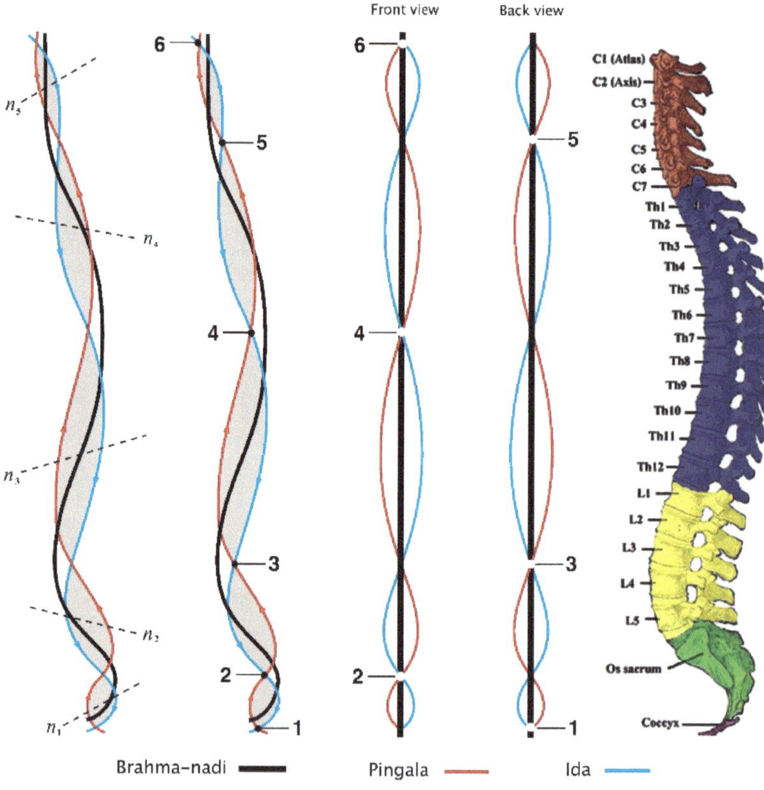

Fig. 5. Central complex. Electromagnetic interactions of 3 main vessels

The loops of spirals of Ida and Pingala cross each other 3 times from 2 sides, forming 5 planes that represent contures of currents. As known, force lines of magnetic field of circuit current pass at 90 angle towards the plane of conductor (Fig. 4) [7]. By this reason Brahma nadi (the flexible magnetic and/or vector 2N (Fig. 3)) curves 5 times towards normal line of each plane, picturing the known contures of central channel of spinal cord (Fig. 5).

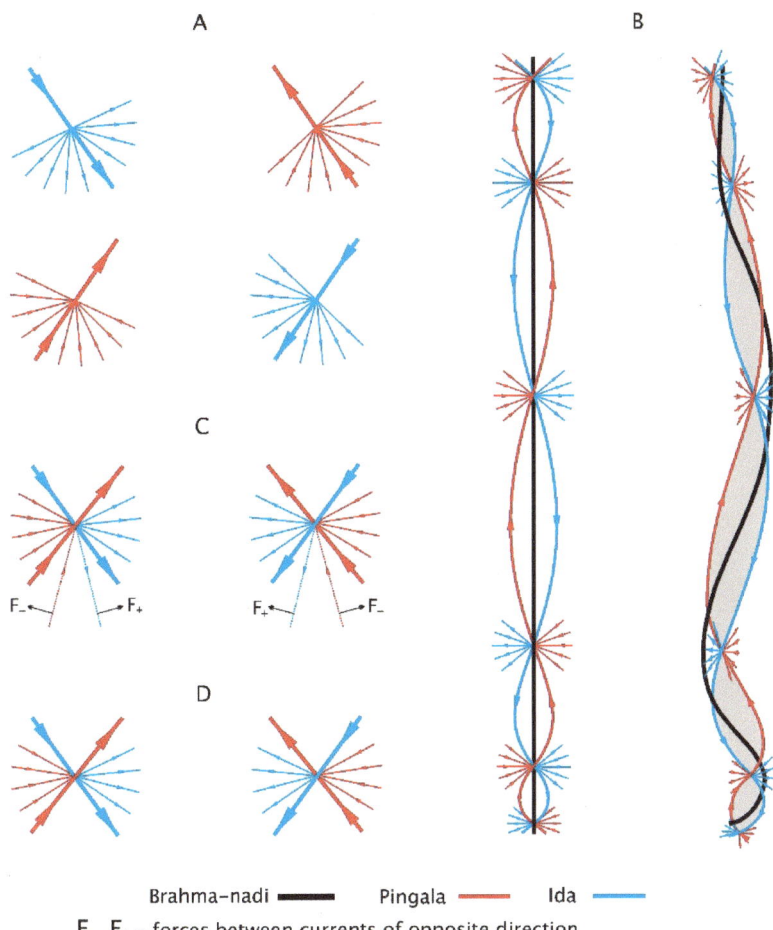

Brahma-nadi ▬▬▬   Pingala ▬▬▬   Ida ▬▬▬
F_−, F_+ – forces between currents of opposite direction

Fig. 6. Separation of Ida and Pingala

Formation of chakras begins from the process of Ida and Pingala separation at the points where they cross each other, when these 2 vessels pass on some distance from each other : as known if currents are in the same direction, they are attracted to each other, and they repel if they are in opposite direction. Newly formed branches (petal vessels or petals) grow to direction of vortex generating them (Fig. 6A). The closer they come to each other, the stronger are repel forces between petals of Ida nad Pingala (Fig. 6 C), in result of which the area of separation is limited within definite borders (Fig. 6 B, D).

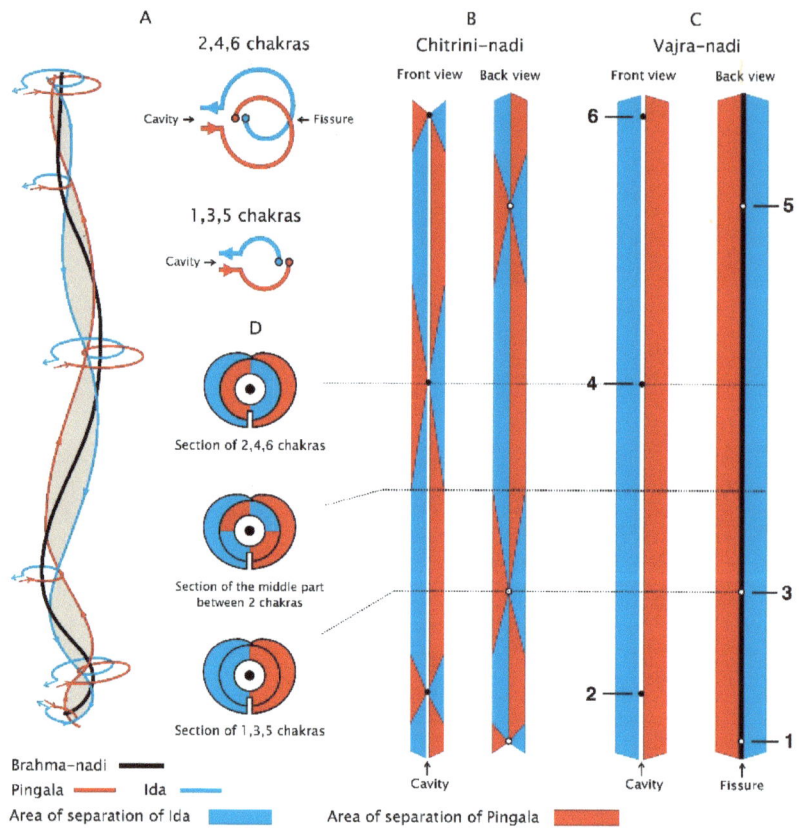

Fig. 7. Formation of Chitrini nadi and Vajra nadi

Later on these "petal vessels" embrace the central complex (Brahma nadi, Ida and Pingala) and meet at the opposite side, forming vessel layer which is coordinated with Chitrini nadi based on sanscript sources. (*all 6 lotos petals are connected to Chitrini nadi*" tc)(Fig. 7A,B). Vajra nadi is formed by petals of 2,4,6 chakras, that embrace the central complex secondary time and meet at front middle line (Fig. 7 A,C). At the same moment right along the line of vessels' transfer from the first layer (Chitrini) into the second one (Vajra) a fissure is coming out, the projection of which to the spinal brain is associated with the backside middle fissure (Fig. 7A). The vessels of polar currents meet at the front middle line, repel each other and create space at the front side as a cavity in the spinal brain to exit out of Sushumna.(Fig. 7 A,C,D).

Later on these vessels make branches and spread all over the body to reach it's surface as acupuncture and biologically active points.

The right side of Vajra nadi consists of only Ida vessels, and the left side- of only Pingala vessels; right and left halves of Chitrini nadi have the equal number of Ida and Pingala petals (Fig. 7B,C). In summary we came to the conclusion that right half is dominated by Ida vessels, and left side – by Pingala vessels (traditionally, the right half of the body is considered to be of masculine origin, and the left side - of feminine one).

On Fig. 5-7 we can see that chakras 2,4,6 are located along frontside of Brahma nadi, and 1,3,5 chakras- along the backside (the sign of opposite), therefore 2,4, 6 chakras are yin, and 1,3,5 are yang. Assuming that yin meridians originate from yin chakras, and yang meridians – from yang chakras and taking into consideration all above factors, we can represent the interconnection of 2 systems in Table 4.

Table 4. 6 main chakras and 12 acupuncture channels

Chakra		Acupuncture channel
1	Muladhara	Stomach and small intestine ST , SI
2	Svadhisthana	Heart, Spleen HT, SP
3	Manipura	Gall bladder and large intestine GB, LI
4	Anahata	Liver and lungs LR, LU
5	Visuddha	Ur. Bladder and 3 heaters BL, TE
6	Ajna	Kidney and pericardium KI, PC

Fig. 8 Kundalini, 3 main nadis (8 A,B) and analog details of given model (section of Sushumna on the level of 1,3,5 chakras and central complex) Fig. 8C.

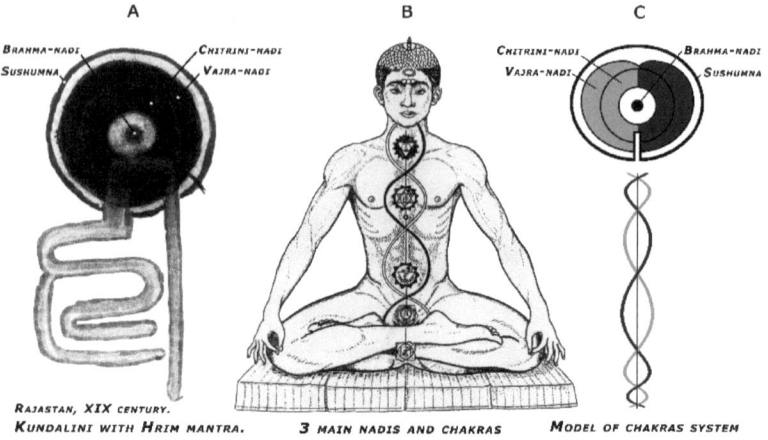

Fig. 8. Sushumna

CONCLUSIONS

1. The concept of yin and yang is applicable to the chakras system as well.
2. Chakras, nadis, acupuncture channels and biologically active points are an integral part of the whole vessel system (*thin or etheric body*).
3. Vital energy (prana or tsi) that circulates through invisible vessels of *thin body* has electromagnetic features.
4. Forms of rough body (in particular, forms of spinal brain and spinal cord) are predetermined by electric processes of the *thin body*.

REFERENCES

1. Atlas of Tibetan Medicine. Collection of illustrations to the medical treatise of 17 century. 1998, p. 100 (in Russian).
2. Adgeat Mukerdji - Kundalini, Arthur Avalon - The Serpent Power. 1997, p.p. 214, 223, 224, 282 (in Russian).
3. Eliade M - Yoga: immortality and freedom. www.gumer.info
4. Chzhud- shek - A monument of Tibetan medieval culture. 1988, p. 30 (in Russian).
5. T. U. Bako, S. G. Gabrielyan,. A Common Theory of Oriental Medicine. An Integral Model for the System of Acupuncture Channels. Collection of articles, 2013 (in Russian). http://www.becomodel.com/, http://www.rusphysics.ru/.
6. Paul P.V. Theory of electricity, 1962, p. 19 (in Russian).
7. Koshkin N.I., Shirkevich M.G. Reference of elementary physics. 1976, p. 155 (in Russian).

Temur Bako (1946 - 2008) graduated from Yerevan State Institute of Physical Culture (1966 – 1971).
From 1988 - 2008 г. he worked on the theme such as *Model of Etheric Physiological Structure of the Body and Methodology of Bio Energy Correlation of Organism (BECO)*.

Susanna Gabrielyan (1960) graduated from Yerevan Polytechnics Institute (1977 – 1982).
From 1992 - present she is engaged with research theme such as *Model of Physiological Structure of the Body and BECO*.

They collaborated with the Laboratory Of Physiology of CNS function compensation, Orbeli Institute of Physiology L.A. Orbelli NAS RA, Clinics of Traditional and Alternative Medicine of National Health Care Institute RA, Science and Medical fund 'Arevelk-Arevmutk'. A research device had been developed to register reactions of the body to the external action via RYO-DO-RAKU points.

HISTORY

LETTER TO CHRISTOPHER RIVE

Dear Mr. Christopher Rive.

I am Mr. Bako Temur (58 years old, higher education in sport medicine). Almost for 15 years I am busy with a scientific work, which directly refers the patients with spinal traumas. I wished to refer this letter to you since 1996 when I read the article about you in the magazine "Sovershenno Secretno" (Top Secret). I was shocked to hear how a very spiritual person could stand such situation. I am carefully keeping the magazine up to now (I am sending the copy to you). I have not seen films with your participation, but I liked you as an individual and I refer to you with sincere respect. Later I wanted to write to support you and inform that practical and scientific research activities are carried out in Armenia in the field of rehabilitation of such patients. I am writing you with delay as far as very lately two scientific articles were published relevant to the theoretical basis of the methodology, that we called bioenergetical correlation of organism. This letter is a revelation about a story that I suppose might interest you.

After the terrible earthquake in Armenia in 1998 there were many patients with spinal traumas who I wanted to be helpful. Before, in 70th worked for physiological institute named after L. A. Orbelli. To my insistent request my friend Mr. John Sarkissian, Doctor of Biological sciences, chief of the Lab. Of Physiology of CNS function compensation, Orbeli Institute of Physiology organized and involved me in the group supporting people who suffered natural disasters. The group worked at the Institute of Phisiology (rehabilitation). Fortunately I could help many of this people thanks to my natural gift (biological background), which I inherited from my forefather physician.

After my approach, the patients sensed currency and pulsations in spinal and lower extremities. In 30-35 days were sensible, after slightly could move first toes and after feet. The patients also felt inch around the abdominal cavity that confirms improvement of digestion and urine-genital functions of the organism. Further we succeed in remarkable increasing the amplitude of motions of extremities. For above mentioned the method of electro stimulation (N- reflexometer), with the help of French hospital apparatus "Alvar".

Taking into consideration the results achieved, physiology Institute administration decided to create a scientific-research group in charge of J. Sarkissian to study the phenomena and improve the methodology of treatment. But in addition to it I aimed in creating an apparatus (kind of biological background strengthener), with the help of which, those without healing gift could cure people as well. Vladimir Avetisyan assisted me in the work, who worked for Institute then.

Since the first day he was the onlooker of my start and feeling inspired with the results of the treatment, created one of the first instrument that fastened the process of rehabilitation up to 20-25 days with 35-40 seconds duration. During the performance many had the feeling of pleasure and asked to lengthen the duration.

I always remember V. Avetisyan with special warmth and merely I cannot forget him rolling 4 000 thin copper cord on toroid core of the apparatus. Presently he lives in the USA.

Unfortunately the plan of creating scientific-research group remained unrealized connected with the fall of the USSR.

The newly created Armenia was not up to science, while there were the times of cold, starvation and poorness, when there was 2 hours electricity per day, one after the other scientific institutions were closing and people selling their housed and leaving abroad.

I remained alone with my dream and ideas, until I met a faithful friend and companion in arms Susanna Gabrielyan. Together with her we created a list of apparatus all by ourselves (shy is a cybernetic with a diploma with honor). Together we also managed in composing our ideas common to scientific language.

As a result cumulative sample of ether-physiological structure of organism, which is the bases of the above mentioned treatment methodology and describes the ether and thin body composition. The governmental attitude towards sciences remained the same and our efforts to bring the idea to life so that it could be the common property of Armenia are destined to fail.

We kept faithful to our ideas, though finally lost any hope that the "Laboratory of Central Nervous System Functions Compensation Physiology" will ever be financed. We did not become members of this laboratory (still keeping in touch with it throughout all these years) as still reduction of positions is continuing at the Institute, the Institute that used to be one of the leading ones in human brains studies during the USSR. Chair of the laboratory J. Sarkissian cannot offer us anything but scientific degrees, which we refused as far as not to draw away from our goal. This is the reason that made us search for support not in Armenia only. You are the firs who I thought of and I am applying to. While searching for your address on the net we were nicely surprised to see your fund is financing as well as scientific researches.

If I try briefly to interpret the plot of energy-correlation method of treatment, then it is rehabilitating the energetic harmony in ether structure of organism that positively influences generally on physical processes and encourages recovery (this principle of treatment is the bases of oriental medicine). The unequal nature of this methodology is that some elements of spiritual practice of yoga is suggested to instilled in medicine (we design to realize it through technical means and physician-bio donor), as well as relieve the potential of oriental reflex therapy through the proposed model of system of meridians. But before we should solve two theoretical problems.

Discoed regularity of energy spread in chakras (special energetic centers located along spinal) and accomplish working out the model of meridians (energetic communication ways).

The suggested method of treatment will be as follows: if earlier during treatment with the first devices I had to intuitively choose bioresonance frequencies of patients, then in future a new device should itself define resonance frequencies of patient at the moment whit the help of biological feedback and to give out definite sequence of frequencies, which should correspond to vibrations of bidja mantras (sound vibrations, by which chakras are characterized). We suppose that it is the bioresonance that makes system of chakras active and ready to accept bioenergy of a donor-healer. Further, energy from system of chakras is distributed through energetic channels (meridians) all over the body. For intensification of healing effect, we suggest to apply Chinese acupuncture based on the new model of meridians, which can scientifically expand opportunities of this ancient medicinal tradition, keeping it's century principles. And definition of functional interconnections of both chakras and meridians can serve as the basis for introduction into reflexotherapy of new methods of treatment, taking into account individual frequency characteristics of the organism.

Positive changes in ether structures reflect on the physical level and bring to recovery. On my opinion, this very event took place in many cases in the past, when patients whit spinal traumas could feel apprehensibility and do some movements because non-conductive tissue scar in injured region of spine became conductive. We believe that changes in this thin ether structures are the reason of all this. We also consider that system of chacres is the more powerful energetic key factor of influence on the organism in comparison with acupuncture channels, this is why this core structure of ether physiology was and remains our main target, to which we aim over 15 years.

On this way we faced the necessity of theoretical basics of Chins medicine. The unexpected result of this a graphic model of system of acupuncture channels, which does not contradict to the well known theory of meridians, but expand it creating more integrated picture of energetic communications of the organism. The model is to be worked out. But inspire this we hope that acupuncture experts will take practical interest to this right today.

Please find enclosed translations of 2 articles in English, which were published in the collection of scientific articles "Information technologies and management" Yerevan № 2-2, 2003 and № 3, 2003.

Sincerely yours
T. Bako